Lynne Robinson is a leading Pilates specialist, whose best-selling first book with Gordon Thomson, *Body Control – The Pilates Way*, has won wide acclaim. Widely featured on TV and in magazines for her work, she is also co-author with Helge Fisher of *Mind-Body Workout*, and is presenter of Telstar's top-selling *Body Control* video, and the new *Pilates Weekly Workout*.

Gordon Thompson, formerly of the Ballet Rambert and London Contemporary Dance, runs the prestigious Body Control Pilates Studio in London's South Kensington. He is co-author of the original *Body Control – The Pilates Way*.

Helge Fisher is qualified in anatomy, physiology and holistic massage, and is an Alexander Technique teacher. The co-author with Lynne Robinson of *Mind-Body Workout*, she has been teaching Body Control Pilates for over ten years.

Advice to the Reader

Before following any of the exercise advice contained in this book it is recommended that you consult your doctor if you suffer from any health problems or special conditions or are in any doubt as to its suitability.

The Desk Reviver

Lynne Robinson, Gordon Thomson & Helge Fisher

PAN BOOKS

First published 1999 by Pan Books

an imprint of Macmillan Publishers Limited
25 Eccleston Place, London SW1W 9NF
and Basingstoke

Associated companies throughout the world

ISBN 0 330 37328 5

9 8 7 6 5 4 3 2 1

A CIP catalogue record for this book is available from the British Library.

Text design by Neil Lang
Printed and bound in Belgium

Contents

Introduction

What a morning! The phone hasn't stopped, you've been stuck at your desk since nine, your shoulders ache, you can feel a tension headache coming on . . .

It's lunchtime, you haven't got time to go to a gym, but you feel sluggish and know that it's going to take more than an egg mayo and cappuccino to revive you.

The following Pilates exercises will reach every part of your body. They'll clear your mind, stretch you out and work those important key muscles, reversing the effects of sitting hunched over the desk all day.

The perfect lunch-break workout, designed so that you can easily exercise in the office with minimal embarrassment and disruption. Just keep a tennis ball and a scarf in the filing cabinet!

The Eight Principles of the Pilates Method

The exercises in this book have their origins in the work of Joseph Pilates (1880–1967). A well proven method in existence for over seventy-five years, they also incorporate the latest techniques in both mental and physical training, offering complete body conditioning.

The programme targets the key postural muscles, building strength from within, by stabilizing the torso. The body is gently realigned and reshaped, the muscles balanced, so that the whole body moves efficiently. By bringing together body and mind and heightening body awareness, Pilates literally teaches you to be in control of your body, allowing you to handle stress more effectively and achieve relaxation more easily.

All the exercises are built around the following Eight Principles:

Relaxation	**Co-ordination**
Concentration	**Centring**
Alignment	**Flowing movements**
Breathing	**Stamina**

Before You Begin

▷ Wear something warm and comfortable, allowing free movement
▷ Slip your shoes off
▷ Keep a long scarf and a tennis ball handy

Please do not exercise if:

▷ You are feeling unwell
▷ You have just eaten your sandwiches
▷ You have a bad hangover
▷ You have taken painkillers, as it will mask any warning pains

If you are undergoing medical treatment, are pregnant or injured, please consult your medical practitioner. It is always advisable to consult your doctor before you take up a new exercise regime.

Checking Your Alignment

Always take a moment to check that your body is correctly aligned before you start an exercise. Here is a checklist to help:

▷ Is my pelvis in neutral? See page 10.
▷ Is my spine lengthened, but still with its natural curves? Think of the top of the head lengthening away from the tailbone.
▷ Where are my shoulders? Hopefully not up around your ears! Keep the shoulder blades down into your back, a nice big gap between the ears and the shoulders.
▷ Is my neck tense? Keep the neck released and soft, the back of the neck stays long.
▷ Where are my feet? Don't forget them, for if they are misplaced it will affect your knees, hips and back. Usually, they should be hip-width apart, in parallel. Watch that they do not roll in or out!

The Position of the Pelvis and Spine

If you exercise with the pelvis and the spine misplaced you run the risk of creating muscle imbalances and stressing the spine itself. You should aim to have your pelvis and spine in their natural, neutral positions.

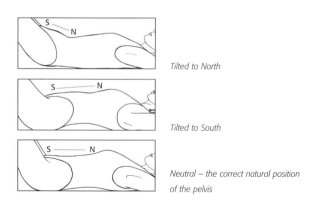

Tilted to North

Tilted to South

Neutral – the correct natural position of the pelvis

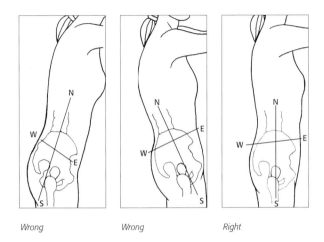

Wrong   *Wrong*   *Right*

Breathing the Pilates Way

In Pilates we use lateral, thoracic breathing for all exercises. This entails breathing into the lower ribcage and back to make maximum use of lung capacity. The increased oxygen intake replenishes the body and the action itself creates greater flexibility in the upper body. It also works the abdominals.

To learn lateral breathing you may sit, stand or kneel, your pelvis in neutral, the spine lengthened.

Wrap a scarf around your ribcage, cross the ends over in the front and pull a little on them to feel where you are working. The idea is to breathe into the scarf, directing the breath into your sides and back, but keeping the shoulders down and relaxed, and the neck calm.

The ribs expand as you inhale, close down as you exhale.

Repeat six times but do not over-breathe or you may feel dizzy.

Breathe softly in a relaxed way.

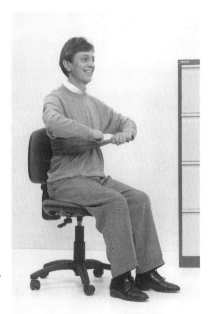

Breathe in wide and
   full to prepare for
      movement
Breathe out as you move
Breathe in to recover

Creating a Strong Centre

Nearly all Pilates exercises involve engaging the deep postural muscles to protect the spine as you exercise. This is called 'stabilizing' or 'centring' and creates a 'girdle of strength' from which to move.

To find these deep muscles, adopt the Starting Position opposite.

▷ Breathe in to prepare and lengthen through the spine.
▷ Breathe out and engage the muscles of your pelvic floor (as if you are trying not to pass water) and hollow your lower abdominals back to your spine. Do not move the pelvis or spine.
▷ Breathe in and release.

Think of it as an internal zip which begins underneath and zips up and in to hold your lower abdominal contents in place, just like zipping up your trousers. '**Zip up and hollow**'.

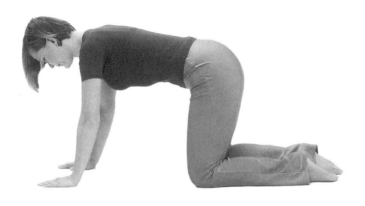

If the office is empty, come onto all fours, hands beneath shoulders, knees beneath your hips. Look straight down at the floor, back of the neck stays long, the spine maintains its natural neutral curve.

If this position is awkward, try 'Zip and Hollow' on page 18.

Grounding While Sitting

Slip your shoes off. Sit with your legs hip-width apart, close to the edge of the chair, your toes parallel. Let your hands rest on your thighs and maintain a neutral pelvis. Release your neck and let the back lengthen.

▷ Be aware of your feet, let them widen and melt into the floor.
▷ Imagine you are growing roots from your toes.
▷ Release tension in your hip joint by gently moving your knees from side to side.
▷ Nod your head.

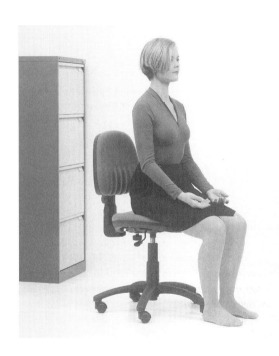

Zip Up and Hollow

Starting Position

Stay in the same position as for 'Grounding while Sitting'. Keep the natural curves of your spine and check that your pelvis is in its neutral position.

Action

This exercise is internal, only slightly visible from the outside. It is another way of isolating the deep-core stabilizing muscles which protect the spine.

▷ Breathe in to prepare and lengthen up through the spine.
▷ Breathe out and engage the muscles of your pelvic floor, as if you are trying to stop the flow of urine, then draw your lower abdominals back towards your spine, **hollowing**. Do not change the alignment of your pelvis and back. Imagine you are '**zipping**' the muscles from the pubic bone up to the navel – as if you were getting into a pair of jeans that are too tight!

▷ Breathe in and release.

Repeat ten times. Keep smiling and no one will know.

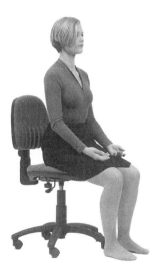

Ankle Circles

Starting Position

Sit with your legs hip-width apart, keeping a long back with its natural curves. Cradle your left thigh with both hands. The right leg stays firmly planted on the floor.

Action

▷ Breathe in and lengthen up through the spine.

▷ Breathe out, zip up and hollow, now straighten the left leg, but be sure not to let your pelvis tilt backwards.

▷ Breathing normally now, circle the ankle slowly inwards, keeping the knees still. Feel the whole foot moving, not just the toes.

Repeat ten times in both directions, with both legs, the slower the better.

Really feel the movement and the muscle action in your legs.

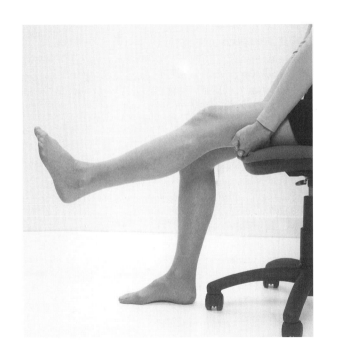

Point and Flex

Starting Position
As for the previous exercise, the hands placed under the right thigh. Spine and pelvis in neutral.

Action
▷ Breathe in and lengthen up through the spine.
▷ Breathe out, **zip up and hollow**, and straighten the right leg, making sure that you do not tip backwards.
▷ Breathing normally now, flex your foot by pushing your heel away from your face, the toes will come towards you. Feel the length down the back of your leg. Then point the toes away from you, keeping them long.

Repeat ten times with each leg, making sure that only the foot, and not the knee, moves and that you keep lengthening up through the spine.

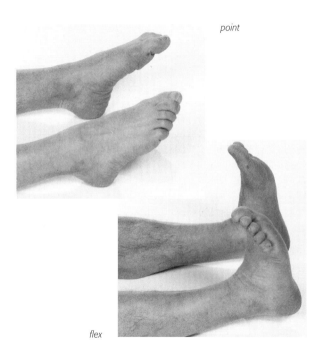

point

flex

Side Reaches

Starting Position

You'll need to turn your chair around for this one. It should be a sturdy chair so, if necessary, borrow your boss's. If you can, sit astride the chair, holding onto the backrest, both sitting bones firmly planted on the chair, your feet flat on the ground.

Please note:

Before doing this exercise, please consult your practitioner if you have a disc-related injury.

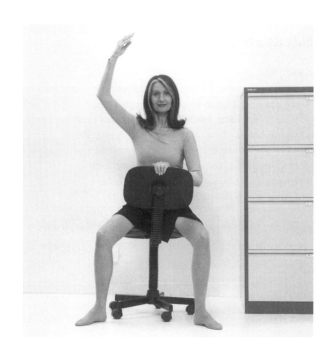

Side Reaches (continued)

Action

▷ Raise one hand over your head, the palm facing downward.

▷ Breathe in and lengthen up through the spine.

▷ Breathe out, **zip up and hollow**, as you slowly reach across to the top corner of the room. Keep your bottom firmly planted while you lift out of the hips. Do not arch your lower back, keep your head and neck in line with the spine.

▷ Breathe in and return to centre, lower the arm.

▷ Change hands and repeat on the other side.

Repeat five times to each side, making sure that you go directly to the side as if moving between two glass doors.

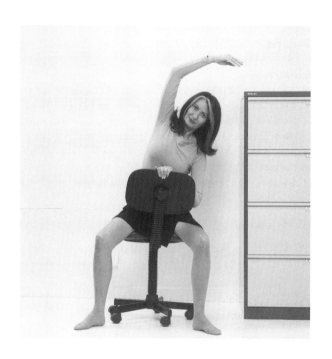

Twister

Starting Position

▷ Sit close to the edge of your chair, your feet firmly planted hip-width apart on the floor. Fold your arms in front of you, in line with your chest.

▷ Keep the shoulders down and your neck soft.

Please note:

Before doing this exercise, please consult your practitioner if you have a disc-related injury.

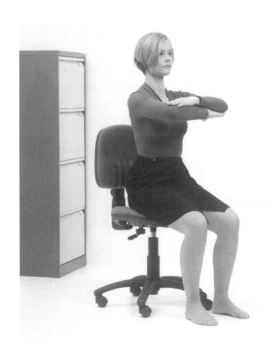

Twister (continued)

Action

▷ Breathe in and lengthen up through your spine.

▷ Breathe out, **zip up and hollow**, and turn to the right as far as you can while keeping your pelvis square and forward facing. Your arms stay at chest height.

▷ Breathe in to lengthen up, still **zipping and hollowing** and return to the front.

Repeat five times to each side. Remember to keep lengthening up.

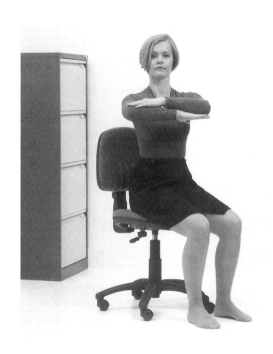

Triceps Stretch

Starting Position

Sit or stand with your pelvis in neutral. Place one hand on the back of your head, at the top of your spine, the other hand at the base of the spine. Keep a sense of openness in the front of your body, but do not allow the back to arch.

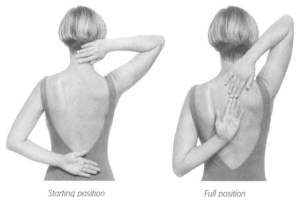

Starting position   *Full position*

Action

▷ Breathe in to prepare and lengthen up through the spine.

▷ Breathe out, **zip up and hollow**, and start tracing the spine
with your fingers until both hands meet. Quite probably
they will not be able to meet – please do not force them!
Do not allow your upper back to arch.

▷ Take two deep breaths, keeping your head central and your
ribs wide.

▷ Breathe out, **zip and hollow**, and slowly trace your spine as
you take your arms back to the starting position.

Repeat three times on each side. It is common for one side to be
harder than the other. If you have your scarf with you, you can
hold on to each end to bring the hands closer – but never strain.

The Dumb Waiter

Starting Position

▷ Sit towards the edge of the
chair, your feet hip-width
apart.

▷ Bring your forearms up to
90-degree angle in front of
your torso, your palms facing
up to the ceiling, your upper
arms along your torso.
Shoulders relaxed, keep the
spine long. Your elbows are
tucked into your waist.

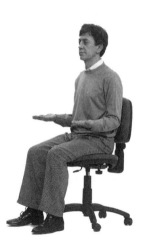

Action

▷ Breathe in and lengthen up through the spine.

▷ Breathe out, **zip up and hollow**.

▷ Breathe in and open your forearms to the sides, keeping the arms parallel with the floor and your elbows close to you. Feel your shoulder blades coming together, keeping them down into your back. Do not allow the back to arch or round.

▷ Breathe in and return to the starting position.

Repeat eight times.

Wrists, Palms and Fingers

Starting Position.

▷ Stand comfortably with your feet hip-width apart and in parallel, your weight evenly balanced on both feet. Check that you are not rolling your feet in or out.

▷ Soft knees.

▷ Find your neutral pelvis position but keep the tailbone lengthening down.

▷ **Zip up and hollow**.

▷ Lengthen up through the top of your head.

▷ Shoulders widening.

▷ Arms relaxing.

Action

▷ Breathe in and lengthen up through the spine.

▷ Breathe out, **zip up and hollow**, bend the elbows and flex the hands towards you, pushing through the wrists, the heel of the hand, the palms and fingers as if you are pushing through water.

▷ Breathe in and return to the starting position.

Repeat eight times, keeping your shoulders down and the movement smooth and flowing.

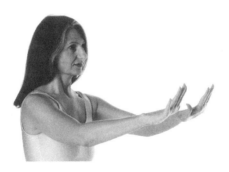

Tennis Ball Exercise

Starting Position
Stand sideways by the cabinet and place the tennis ball between your ankles, just below your inside ankle bone. Hold onto the cabinet.

Action
▷ Breathe in and lengthen up through the spine – imagine someone is pulling you up from the top of your head, but that there is also a weight on your tailbone, anchoring your spine.

▷ Breathe out, **zipping up and hollowing**, and rise up onto your toes.

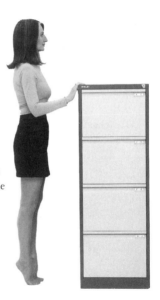

▷ Breathe in.

▷ Breathe out, and slowly lengthen your heels back down on the floor away from the top of your head. Imagine that your head stays up there.

▷ When your heels are on the floor, breathe in and out and slightly bend your knees directly over your feet, keeping the heels down. Do not allow your bottom to stick out.

▷ Straighten your legs.

Repeat ten times.

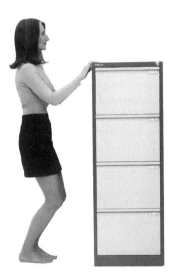

One-legged Cabinet Exercise

These cabinet exercises are a super workout for the legs. Who needs to go to the gym?

Starting Position
Still standing by the cabinet, discard the tennis ball – with some consideration to your fellow employees, please! Bend one leg so that the knee faces straight forward and the foot is resting just beside the other knee. Hold onto the cabinet.

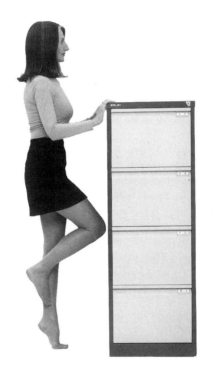

One-legged Cabinet Exercise

Action
▷ Breathe in and lengthen up through the spine.
▷ Breathe out, **zip up and hollow**, and rise up onto your toes.
▷ Breathe in.
▷ Breathe out and slowly lower the heel back down on the floor away from the top of your hand.
▷ Breathe in when the heel has landed.
▷ Breathe out, **zip and hollow**, bend your knee, bringing the knee cap directly over the centre of your foot. As you do so, do not sink into your hips, keep lengthening up and keep your pelvis level.
▷ Breathe in and straighten the leg.

Repeat five times on each leg. Do not allow your bottom to stick out. Think of the weight on your tailbone.

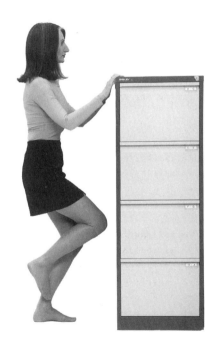

Roll Downs on the Wall

A wonderful exercise for making the spine flexible and strong. It is also great for releasing tension in the neck, arms and shoulders – as rejuvenating as a long weekend break!

Please note:
If you have a back injury, please take advice from your specialist before doing this exercise.

Starting Position
Stand with your feet about forty-five centimetres from a wall, hip-width apart and in parallel. Lean back into the wall bending the knees – if viewed from the side, you will look as though you are sitting on a high stool. Don't try to take your head back onto the wall.

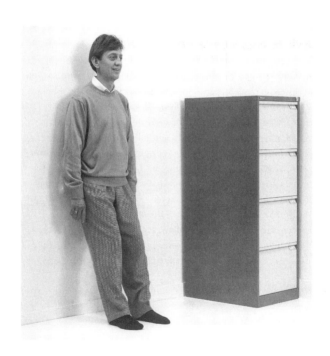

Roll Downs on the Wall (continued)

Action

▷ Breathe in to prepare and lengthen up through the spine.

▷ Breathe out, **zip up and hollow**, allow the chin to drop forward by letting go of the head and neck. Allow the weight of your head to help you roll forward.

▷ Peel the spine off the wall. Your neck, arms and hands are relaxed. Your bottom remains on the wall. Only go as far as you are comfortable but aim to reach the floor eventually – you may bend your knees more.

▷ Breathe in as you hang, keep **zipping and hollowing**.

▷ Breathe out, **zip up and hollow**, rotate the pelvis backwards, bringing the pubic bone toward the chin, slowly bone by bone curl your spine back onto the wall as you come up.

Repeat six times, wheeling the spine and 'working out' any stiff areas.

Remember to breathe out as you move the spine.

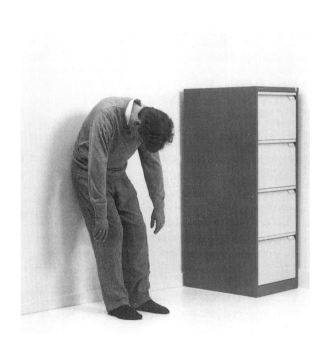